Herbal Remedies for Women

A Complete Guide to Natural Healing with Herbs, Essential Oils, and Tinctures for Hormonal Balance, Stress Relief, and Vitality

Ilera Loro

Copyright © 2024 by Ilera Loro

Disclaimer

The information in "**Herbal Remedies for Women**" is intended for educational purposes only and is not a substitute for professional medical advice, diagnosis, or treatment. Always consult with a qualified healthcare provider before starting any new health regimen, especially if you are **pregnant, nursing, have a medical condition, or are taking medication.** The author and publisher are not responsible for any adverse effects or consequences resulting from the use of the information contained in this book.

Table of Contents

Introduction
The Power of Herbal Remedies

Herbal remedies have been cherished for centuries across cultures for their healing properties and natural efficacy. These remedies, derived from plants, offer a gentle yet powerful approach to health and wellness. Unlike many synthetic medications, herbs work harmoniously with our bodies, supporting natural processes and fostering overall well-being. By tapping into the power of herbs, we can address a wide range of health issues with fewer side effects and a holistic touch.

Why Focus on Women's Health?

Women's bodies are wonderfully complex, with unique needs and rhythms. From menstrual cycles and pregnancy to menopause and beyond, women's health journeys are deeply influenced by hormonal changes. This book focuses on women's health to provide targeted support for these distinct phases of life. By understanding and addressing these unique needs, we can enhance our quality of life, boost vitality, and promote long-term wellness.

Understanding Hormonal Balance, Stress Relief, and Vitality

Hormonal balance is crucial for women's health, impacting everything from mood and energy levels to reproductive health. When hormones are out of sync, it can lead to a variety of issues such as irregular periods, mood swings, and fatigue. This book offers natural solutions to help restore balance and harmony within your body.

Stress is an inevitable part of life, but it doesn't have to control us. Chronic stress can have a detrimental effect on both physical and mental health. Herbal remedies provide a natural way to manage stress, soothe the mind, and support the body's stress response.

Vitality goes beyond mere absence of disease; it's about thriving and feeling vibrant at every stage of life. Through the right combination of herbs, essential oils, and lifestyle practices, you can boost your energy levels, enhance your resilience, and embrace life with zest and enthusiasm.

How to Use This Book

This book is designed to be a comprehensive guide to natural healing with herbs, essential oils, and tinctures, tailored specifically for women. Each chapter delves into different aspects of women's health, offering detailed information on various herbs and their uses. You'll find practical tips, easy-to-follow recipes, and insightful advice to help you incorporate these natural remedies into your daily routine.

Whether you're a beginner looking to explore herbal remedies or someone with some experience seeking deeper knowledge, this book has something for you. Use it as a reference guide, a source of inspiration, and a companion on your journey to natural health and vitality. Each chapter builds on the previous one, creating a cohesive and comprehensive approach to women's wellness. Embrace the wisdom of nature and empower yourself to take charge of your health with the nurturing power of herbs.

Chapter 1:
The Basics of Herbal Medicine

History of Herbal Remedies

Herbal medicine is one of the oldest forms of healing, with roots stretching back to ancient civilizations. Cultures around the world have relied on plants to treat ailments and maintain health, passing down their knowledge through generations.

Ancient Civilizations:

- **Egyptians**: The Egyptians documented their use of herbs as far back as 1500 BCE in texts such as the Ebers Papyrus, which lists over 700 medicinal substances derived from plants.

- **Chinese**: Traditional Chinese Medicine (TCM) has a history of over 2,000 years, with foundational texts like the "Shennong Bencao Jing" detailing the therapeutic properties of various herbs.

- **Indians**: Ayurveda, the ancient Indian system of medicine, extensively uses herbs. Texts such as the "Charaka Samhita" and "Sushruta Samhita" highlight numerous herbal treatments.

- **Greeks and Romans**: Hippocrates and Galen, prominent figures in ancient Greek and Roman medicine, advocated for the use of herbs in treating diseases, influencing Western herbal practices for centuries.

Medieval Europe: During the Middle Ages, monastic gardens flourished with medicinal herbs. Monks and nuns preserved ancient texts and contributed their knowledge, forming the basis for modern Western herbalism.

Indigenous Cultures: Native American, African, and other indigenous cultures also developed rich herbal traditions, often based on the local flora. These cultures view plants as integral to their spiritual and physical well-being.

Modern Herbalism: The 19th and 20th centuries saw a decline in herbal medicine with the rise of synthetic pharmaceuticals. However, there has been a resurgence in recent decades as people seek natural and holistic approaches to health.

Understanding Herbs, Essential Oils, and Tinctures

Herbs: Herbs are plants or plant parts valued for their medicinal, aromatic, or savory qualities. They can be used fresh or dried, and different parts of the plant (leaves, flowers, roots, seeds) may be utilized depending on the herb and its intended use.

- **Infusions and Decoctions**: Infusions are made by steeping herbs in hot water, similar to making tea, ideal for delicate parts like leaves and flowers. Decoctions involve simmering tougher parts like roots and bark to extract their benefits.

Essential Oils: Essential oils are concentrated extracts from aromatic plants. They capture the plant's scent and volatile compounds, offering therapeutic benefits through inhalation or topical application.

- **Extraction Methods**: Steam distillation and cold pressing are common methods. Essential oils should always be diluted in a carrier oil before applying to the skin to avoid irritation.

Tinctures: Tinctures are potent liquid extracts made by soaking herbs in alcohol or vinegar. This method preserves the active constituents of the herb and has a long shelf life.

- **Preparation**: To make a tincture, combine dried or fresh herbs with alcohol (usually vodka or brandy) in a jar. Let it sit for several weeks, shaking occasionally. Strain out the plant material and store the liquid in a dark bottle.

How Herbs Work in the Body

Herbs interact with the body in various ways to promote healing and wellness. Here are some mechanisms through which herbs exert their effects:

Phytochemicals: Herbs contain bioactive compounds known as phytochemicals, which have therapeutic properties. Examples include flavonoids, alkaloids, terpenes, and polyphenols. These compounds can act as antioxidants, anti-inflammatories, antimicrobials, and more.

Synergy: Unlike synthetic drugs, herbs often contain multiple compounds that work together synergistically. This means the combined effect of these compounds can be greater than the sum of their individual effects.

Adaptogens: Some herbs are classified as adaptogens, meaning they help the body adapt to stress and maintain balance. Examples include ashwagandha, Rhodiola, and Holy Basil.

Nutritional Support: Herbs can provide vitamins, minerals, and other nutrients that support overall health. For instance, nettle is rich in iron, calcium, and magnesium.

Modulation of Bodily Systems: Herbs can influence various bodily systems, such as the endocrine, digestive, nervous, and immune systems. For example, peppermint aids digestion, while valerian root promotes relaxation.

Safety and Precautions

While herbs are natural, it's crucial to use them safely and responsibly. Here are some key considerations:

Quality and Sourcing:

- **Quality**: Always use high-quality herbs from reputable sources to ensure purity and potency. Look for organic, non-GMO, and sustainably harvested products when possible.

- **Sourcing**: Be mindful of the herb's origin. Wildcrafted herbs should be harvested sustainably to avoid depleting natural populations.

Dosage and Administration:

- **Dosage**: Follow recommended dosages and consult with a healthcare provider, especially if you are pregnant, nursing, or taking medications.

- **Administration**: Different herbs and preparations may require specific administration methods for optimal efficacy.

Allergies and Sensitivities:

- Conduct a patch test before using a new essential oil or topical herb to check for allergic reactions.

- Be aware of potential allergic reactions and discontinue use if adverse effects occur.

Interactions with Medications:

- Some herbs can interact with prescription medications, altering their effects. For instance, St. John's Wort can reduce the efficacy of certain drugs, including birth control pills.

- Always consult with a healthcare provider before combining herbs with medications.

Toxicity and Side Effects:

- Some herbs can be toxic in high doses or if used improperly. For example, comfrey should not be taken internally due to potential liver toxicity.

- Be aware of possible side effects and use herbs as recommended.

By understanding the basics of herbal medicine, you can harness the power of nature to support your health and well-being. As you explore the subsequent chapters, you'll gain deeper insights into specific herbs and their applications for women's health, hormonal balance, stress relief, and vitality.

Chapter 2:
Hormonal Balance and Women's Health

Common Hormonal Imbalances in Women

Hormonal imbalances can significantly impact women's health, leading to a range of symptoms and conditions. Hormones are chemical messengers that regulate various bodily functions, including metabolism, mood, reproduction, and growth. Here are some common hormonal imbalances women may experience:

1. Premenstrual Syndrome (PMS) and Premenstrual Dysphoric Disorder (PMDD):

- **Symptoms**: Bloating, mood swings, irritability, fatigue, and breast tenderness.

- **Causes**: Fluctuations in estrogen and progesterone levels during the menstrual cycle.

2. Polycystic Ovary Syndrome (PCOS):

- **Symptoms**: Irregular periods, weight gain, acne, hirsutism (excessive hair growth), and fertility issues.

- **Causes**: Elevated levels of androgens (male hormones) and insulin resistance.

3. Thyroid Disorders:

- **Hypothyroidism**: Low thyroid hormone levels causing fatigue, weight gain, and depression.

- **Hyperthyroidism**: Excessive thyroid hormone levels leading to weight loss, anxiety, and palpitations.

4. Menopause and Perimenopause:

- **Symptoms**: Hot flashes, night sweats, mood swings, vaginal dryness, and sleep disturbances.

- **Causes**: Decrease in estrogen and progesterone production as women age.

5. Estrogen Dominance:

- **Symptoms**: Heavy periods, breast tenderness, fibroids, and weight gain.

- **Causes**: Excessive estrogen relative to progesterone, often due to lifestyle factors and environmental toxins.

6. Adrenal Fatigue:

- **Symptoms**: Chronic fatigue, cravings for salty foods, weakened immunity, and difficulty handling stress.

- **Causes**: Prolonged stress leading to overworked adrenal glands and imbalanced cortisol levels.

Understanding these imbalances and their underlying causes can help women take proactive steps to restore hormonal harmony. Herbal remedies offer a natural and effective approach to managing these conditions.

Herbs for Menstrual Health

Balancing hormones naturally can alleviate many menstrual issues. Here are some key herbs that support menstrual health:

Chasteberry (Vitex agnus-castus):

- **Uses**: Known for its ability to regulate menstrual cycles, reduce PMS symptoms, and support fertility.

- **Mechanism**: Chasteberry works by influencing the pituitary gland to balance the production of progesterone and estrogen.

- **Preparation**: Typically taken as a tincture or capsule. Dosage varies, but a common recommendation is 20-40 mg of dried fruit extract daily.

- **Considerations**: It may take several months to notice significant effects. Consult a healthcare provider if you have hormone-sensitive conditions.

Dong Quai (Angelica sinensis):

- **Uses**: Often referred to as the "female ginseng," Dong Quai is used to alleviate menstrual cramps, regulate cycles, and support overall reproductive health.

- **Mechanism**: Contains phytoestrogens that help balance estrogen levels and improve blood circulation to the pelvic area.

- **Preparation**: Can be consumed as a tea, tincture, or capsule. A typical dose is 1-2 grams of dried root daily.

- **Considerations**: Avoid during pregnancy and if you have heavy menstrual bleeding.

Black Cohosh (Cimicifuga racemosa):

- **Uses**: Effective in reducing menstrual pain, alleviating PMS symptoms, and treating menopausal symptoms.

- **Mechanism**: Contains compounds that mimic estrogen and help regulate hormone levels.

- **Preparation**: Available as a tea, tincture, or capsule. The standard dose is 20-40 mg of standardized extract daily.

- **Considerations**: Consult a healthcare provider before use if you have a history of breast cancer or liver issues.

Herbs for Menopause Relief

Menopause marks a significant hormonal shift, and certain herbs can help ease the transition:

Red Clover (Trifolium pratense):

- **Uses**: Red Clover is used to reduce hot flashes, improve bone density, and support cardiovascular health during menopause.

- **Mechanism**: Rich in isoflavones, which are plant-based compounds that mimic estrogen and help balance hormone levels.

- **Preparation**: Often taken as a tea, tincture, or capsule. A common dose is 40-80 mg of standardized extract daily.

- **Considerations**: Consult a healthcare provider before use if you have a history of hormone-sensitive conditions.

Sage (Salvia officinalis):

- **Uses**: Known for its ability to reduce hot flashes and excessive sweating associated with menopause.

- **Mechanism**: Contains compounds that have estrogenic properties and help regulate body temperature.

- **Preparation**: Commonly consumed as a tea or tincture. A typical dose is 1-4 grams of dried leaves daily or 1-2 teaspoons of tincture.

- **Considerations**: Sage essential oil should not be ingested. Use caution if you have epilepsy or other seizure disorders.

Wild Yam (Dioscorea villosa):

- **Uses**: Wild Yam is used to relieve menopausal symptoms, including hot flashes and vaginal dryness, and support overall hormonal balance.

- **Mechanism**: Contains diosgenin, a compound that can be converted into progesterone in the lab, though the body does not convert it directly.

- **Preparation**: Available as a cream, tincture, or capsule. Topical application is common for menopausal symptom relief.

- **Considerations**: Not all wild yam products are standardized, so choose a reputable brand. Consult a healthcare provider for proper use.

Hormonal imbalances can significantly impact a woman's quality of life, but nature offers a bounty of remedies to help restore balance. By understanding the specific needs of your body and incorporating these herbs into your routine, you can address common issues such as menstrual irregularities, PMS, and menopausal symptoms naturally. As always, it's important to consult with a healthcare provider before starting any new herbal regimen, especially if you have underlying health conditions or are taking other medications. Through informed choices and the power of herbal medicine, you can achieve better hormonal health and overall well-being.

Chapter 3:
Herbal Remedies for Stress Relief
The Impact of Stress on Women's Health

Stress is a ubiquitous part of modern life, but its effects can be particularly pronounced in women due to their unique hormonal cycles and life stages. Chronic stress can lead to a host of health issues, including:

1. Hormonal Imbalances:

- **Disruption of Menstrual Cycle**: Stress can alter the regularity of menstrual cycles, causing missed or irregular periods.

- **Aggravation of PMS and PMDD**: Elevated stress levels can worsen premenstrual symptoms, leading to severe mood swings, irritability, and physical discomfort.

- **Impact on Fertility**: Prolonged stress can interfere with ovulation and reduce the chances of conception.

2. Mental Health:

- **Anxiety and Depression**: Chronic stress is a significant risk factor for developing anxiety and depression. Women are particularly susceptible due to hormonal fluctuations.

- **Cognitive Decline**: Persistent stress can impair memory, focus, and overall cognitive function.

3. Physical Health:

- **Immune System Suppression**: Stress weakens the immune system, making the body more vulnerable to infections and illnesses.

- **Cardiovascular Issues**: Chronic stress increases the risk of hypertension, heart disease, and stroke.

- **Digestive Problems**: Stress can exacerbate conditions like irritable bowel syndrome (IBS), leading to discomfort and digestive disturbances.

Understanding the profound impact of stress on women's health underscores the importance of managing it effectively. Herbal remedies offer a natural and holistic approach to stress relief.

Adaptogenic Herbs

Adaptogens are a unique class of herbs that help the body adapt to stress, enhance resilience, and maintain balance. They work by modulating the stress response and supporting the adrenal glands.

Ashwagandha (Withania somnifera):

- **Uses**: Ashwagandha is renowned for its ability to reduce stress and anxiety, improve sleep, and enhance overall well-being.

- **Mechanism**: Contains compounds that normalize cortisol levels, the hormone associated with the stress response. It also supports the nervous system and boosts energy.

- **Preparation**: Available as a powder, capsule, or tincture. A typical dose is 300-600 mg of standardized extract taken once or twice daily.

- **Considerations**: Generally safe for long-term use. Consult a healthcare provider if you are pregnant or have autoimmune conditions.

Rhodiola (Rhodiola rosea):

- **Uses**: Rhodiola is effective in reducing fatigue, improving mood, and enhancing mental clarity and physical performance.

- **Mechanism**: Acts by regulating the hypothalamic-pituitary-adrenal (HPA) axis and balancing neurotransmitters like serotonin and dopamine.

- **Preparation**: Commonly taken as a capsule or tincture. The typical dose is 200-600 mg of standardized extract daily, taken in the morning or early afternoon.

- **Considerations**: Can be stimulating for some individuals. Avoid taking it late in the day to prevent insomnia.

Holy Basil (Ocimum sanctum):

- **Uses**: Holy Basil, also known as Tulsi, is used to reduce stress, promote relaxation, and support overall emotional well-being.

- **Mechanism**: Contains compounds that lower cortisol levels and enhance the body's stress resilience. It also has antioxidant and anti-inflammatory properties.

- **Preparation**: Consumed as a tea, capsule, or tincture. A typical dose is 300-600 mg of standardized extract daily or 1-2 cups of tea.

- **Considerations**: Generally safe for long-term use. Consult a healthcare provider if you are pregnant or breastfeeding.

Calming Herbs

Calming herbs help soothe the nervous system, reduce anxiety, and promote relaxation without causing sedation or dependence.

Lavender (Lavandula angustifolia):

- **Uses**: Lavender is widely known for its calming and relaxing effects, making it effective for reducing anxiety and improving sleep quality.

- **Mechanism**: Contains linalool and linalyl acetate, compounds that interact with the neurotransmitter GABA (gamma-aminobutyric acid) to promote relaxation.

- **Preparation**: Used as an essential oil for aromatherapy, as well as in teas and tinctures. For aromatherapy, diffuse a few drops or add to a warm bath. As a tea, steep 1-2 teaspoons of dried flowers in hot water.

- **Considerations**: Generally safe. Avoid ingesting essential oils and consult a healthcare provider before use during pregnancy.

Chamomile (Matricaria chamomilla):

- **Uses**: Chamomile is known for its gentle calming effects, making it ideal for reducing anxiety, improving sleep, and soothing digestive issues.

- **Mechanism**: Contains apigenin, a compound that binds to GABA receptors in the brain, promoting relaxation and reducing anxiety.

- **Preparation**: Commonly consumed as a tea. Steep 1-2 teaspoons of dried flowers in hot water for 5-10 minutes. Also available as capsules and tinctures.

- **Considerations**: Generally safe for most people. Avoid if you have allergies to plants in the Asteraceae family.

Valerian Root (Valeriana officinalis):

- **Uses**: Valerian root is highly effective in reducing anxiety, promoting relaxation, and improving sleep quality.

- **Mechanism**: Enhances the release of GABA in the brain, leading to sedative and anxiolytic effects.

- **Preparation**: Available as a tea, tincture, or capsule. A typical dose is 400-900 mg of standardized extract or 1 teaspoon of tincture taken before bedtime.

- **Considerations**: May cause drowsiness. Avoid operating heavy machinery after use and consult a healthcare provider before long-term use.

Stress is an inevitable part of life, but its impact on women's health can be profound. By incorporating adaptogenic and calming herbs into your daily routine, you can effectively manage stress, enhance resilience, and promote overall well-being. Remember to consult with a healthcare provider before starting any new herbal regimen, especially if you have underlying health conditions or are taking other medications. Through the wisdom of herbal remedies, you can find natural and holistic solutions to stress relief and embrace a healthier, more balanced life.

Chapter 4:
Boosting Vitality and Energy
Understanding Fatigue and Low Energy

Fatigue and low energy are common complaints among women, often stemming from various physical, emotional, and lifestyle factors. Understanding the root causes is essential for addressing these issues effectively:

1. Hormonal Imbalances:

- **Thyroid Issues**: Hypothyroidism can lead to persistent fatigue, weight gain, and depression due to low thyroid hormone levels.

- **Adrenal Fatigue**: Chronic stress can overwork the adrenal glands, leading to imbalanced cortisol levels and feelings of exhaustion.

- **Menstrual Cycle**: Fluctuations in estrogen and progesterone can cause premenstrual fatigue or tiredness during menstruation.

2. Nutritional Deficiencies:

- **Iron Deficiency**: Common in women due to menstruation, iron deficiency can cause anemia, leading to extreme tiredness and weakness.

- **Vitamin B12 and D Deficiency**: These vitamins are crucial for energy production and overall vitality.

3. Lifestyle Factors:

- **Sleep Deprivation**: Poor sleep quality or insufficient sleep can significantly impact energy levels.

- **Diet and Hydration**: A diet lacking in nutrients or inadequate hydration can lead to fatigue.

- **Lack of Physical Activity**: Sedentary lifestyles can decrease energy levels and overall vitality.

4. Mental Health:

- **Stress and Anxiety**: Mental stress and anxiety can drain energy and disrupt sleep, leading to fatigue.

- **Depression**: Fatigue is a common symptom of depression, affecting daily activities and overall quality of life.

Addressing these underlying causes through lifestyle changes and herbal remedies can help boost energy and vitality.

Energizing Herbs

Herbal remedies offer a natural and effective way to boost energy levels and enhance vitality. Here are some key energizing herbs:

Ginseng (Panax ginseng and Panax quinquefolius):

- **Uses**: Ginseng is renowned for its ability to enhance physical and mental performance, reduce fatigue, and improve overall vitality.

- **Mechanism**: Contains ginsenosides, compounds that help reduce oxidative stress, improve mitochondrial function, and enhance the body's resistance to stress.

- **Preparation**: Available as a tea, tincture, or capsule. The typical dose for Panax ginseng (Asian ginseng) is 200-400 mg of standardized extract daily. For Panax quinquefolius (American ginseng), a similar dose is recommended.

- **Considerations**: Can be stimulating, so avoid taking it late in the day. Consult a healthcare provider if you have high blood pressure, diabetes, or are taking other medications.

Maca Root (Lepidium meyenii):

- **Uses**: Maca root is known for boosting energy, enhancing stamina, and supporting hormonal balance.

- **Mechanism**: Rich in vitamins, minerals, and amino acids, maca supports endocrine function and helps maintain optimal energy levels.

- **Preparation**: Typically consumed as a powder added to smoothies, oatmeal, or other foods. A common dose is 1-3 teaspoons daily. Also available in capsule form.

- **Considerations**: Generally safe for long-term use. Start with a lower dose and gradually increase to assess tolerance.

Licorice Root (Glycyrrhiza glabra):

- **Uses**: Licorice root is used to combat fatigue, support adrenal function, and enhance overall vitality.

- **Mechanism**: Contains glycyrrhizin, which helps regulate cortisol levels and supports adrenal health. Also has anti-inflammatory and immune-boosting properties.

- **Preparation**: Available as a tea, tincture, or capsule. A typical dose is 1-2 grams of dried root or 30-60 drops of tincture daily.

- **Considerations**: Prolonged use can lead to elevated blood pressure and reduced potassium levels. Use with caution if you have hypertension or heart disease, and consult a healthcare provider for long-term use.

Daily Vitality Routines

Incorporating energizing herbs into daily routines, along with lifestyle practices, can significantly boost vitality and overall energy levels:

1. Morning Rituals:

- **Herbal Tea or Smoothie**: Start the day with a cup of energizing herbal tea or a smoothie blended with maca powder and ginseng extract.

- **Stretching and Movement**: Engage in gentle stretching or a quick morning exercise routine to stimulate blood flow and wake up the body.

- **Mindfulness Practice**: Spend a few minutes in meditation or deep breathing to set a positive tone for the day and reduce stress.

2. Balanced Nutrition:

- **Nutritious Breakfast**: Include a balanced breakfast rich in protein, healthy fats, and complex carbohydrates to sustain energy levels throughout the day.

- **Hydration**: Drink plenty of water throughout the day to stay hydrated and support overall energy.

3. Midday Boost:

- **Herbal Supplements**: Take a dose of ginseng or licorice root tincture during the mid-afternoon slump to maintain energy levels.

- **Light Exercise**: Incorporate a short walk or light exercise to re-energize and break up sedentary periods.

4. Stress Management:

- **Adaptogenic Herbs**: Incorporate adaptogens like ashwagandha or holy basil to help manage stress and support adrenal health.

- **Relaxation Techniques**: Practice relaxation techniques such as yoga, tai chi, or progressive muscle relaxation to reduce stress and enhance vitality.

5. Evening Wind-Down:

- **Calming Herbal Tea**: End the day with a calming herbal tea like chamomile or lavender to promote relaxation and improve sleep quality.

- **Sleep Hygiene**: Establish a consistent sleep routine, create a restful environment, and aim for 7-9 hours of quality sleep each night.

6. Regular Exercise:

- **Consistency**: Engage in regular physical activity such as walking, swimming, or dancing to boost energy levels and improve overall health.

- **Variety**: Include a mix of cardiovascular, strength, and flexibility exercises to keep the routine enjoyable and comprehensive.

7. Periodic Detoxification:

- **Herbal Detox**: Periodically incorporate detoxifying herbs like dandelion or milk thistle to support liver health and overall vitality.

- **Clean Eating**: Emphasize whole, unprocessed foods and minimize intake of sugar, caffeine, and alcohol.

Boosting vitality and energy is about nurturing your body, mind, and spirit through a holistic approach. By understanding the underlying causes of fatigue and incorporating energizing herbs and healthy lifestyle practices into your daily routine, you can achieve sustained energy levels and enhanced overall well-being. Always consult with a healthcare provider before starting any new herbal regimen, especially if you have underlying health conditions or are taking other medications. Through the natural power of herbal remedies and mindful living, you can embrace a life full of energy and vitality.

Chapter 5:
Herbal Remedies for Skin and Beauty

Common Skin Issues and Their Herbal Solutions

Women often face various skin issues due to hormonal changes, environmental factors, and lifestyle choices. Herbal remedies provide natural and effective solutions for maintaining healthy skin and addressing common concerns.

1. Acne:

- **Causes**: Hormonal imbalances, excess oil production, bacteria, and clogged pores.

- **Herbal Solutions**:

  - **Tea Tree Oil**: Has antibacterial properties that help reduce acne-causing bacteria.

  - **Calendula**: Anti-inflammatory and healing, helps soothe irritated skin.

  - **Aloe Vera**: Reduces inflammation and accelerates healing of acne lesions.

2. Eczema and Dermatitis:

- **Causes**: Allergic reactions, genetic factors, stress, and irritants.

- **Herbal Solutions**:

  - **Chamomile**: Anti-inflammatory and soothing, helps reduce redness and irritation.

  - **Calendula**: Promotes healing and reduces inflammation.

  - **Oatmeal**: Moisturizing and soothing, often used in baths to relieve itching.

3. Dry Skin:

- **Causes**: Environmental factors, dehydration, and aging.

- **Herbal Solutions**:

  - **Aloe Vera**: Hydrates and soothes dry skin.

  - **Coconut Oil**: Moisturizing and protective, helps retain skin moisture.

  - **Lavender**: Calming and moisturizing, also has mild antibacterial properties.

4. Hyperpigmentation:

- **Causes**: Sun exposure, hormonal changes, and skin inflammation.

- **Herbal Solutions**:

  - **Licorice Root**: Contains glabridin, which inhibits melanin production and lightens dark spots.

  - **Turmeric**: Anti-inflammatory and brightening, helps reduce pigmentation.

  - **Aloe Vera**: Promotes healing and lightens dark spots.

5. Aging and Wrinkles:

- **Causes**: Sun exposure, loss of collagen and elastin, and environmental damage.

- **Herbal Solutions**:

  - **Rosehip Oil**: Rich in vitamins A and C, promotes collagen production and skin regeneration.

  - **Green Tea**: Contains antioxidants that protect against UV damage and reduce signs of aging.

o **Ginseng**: Improves skin elasticity and reduces wrinkles.

Herbs for Healthy Skin

Calendula (Calendula officinalis):

- **Uses**: Known for its anti-inflammatory, antiseptic, and healing properties, Calendula is excellent for soothing irritated skin, reducing inflammation, and promoting wound healing.

- **Mechanism**: Contains flavonoids and triterpenoids that reduce inflammation and promote tissue regeneration.

- **Preparation**: Often used as an infused oil, salve, or cream. To make an infused oil, steep dried calendula flowers in carrier oil (such as olive oil) for several weeks.

- **Considerations**: Generally safe for all skin types. Perform a patch test if you have sensitive skin.

Aloe Vera (Aloe barbadensis miller):

- **Uses**: Aloe Vera is renowned for its soothing, hydrating, and healing properties, making it ideal for treating burns, acne, and dry skin.

- **Mechanism**: Contains vitamins, minerals, and polysaccharides that promote skin healing, reduce inflammation, and provide deep hydration.

- **Preparation**: Use the gel directly from the plant or buy pure Aloe Vera gel. Apply to the skin as needed.

- **Considerations**: Generally safe for topical use. Perform a patch test if you have sensitive skin.

Tea Tree Oil (Melaleuca alternifolia):

- **Uses**: Tea Tree Oil is widely used for its antibacterial, antifungal, and anti-inflammatory properties, making it effective against acne, fungal infections, and minor cuts.

- **Mechanism**: Contains terpenes that kill bacteria and fungi, reduce inflammation, and promote healing.

- **Preparation**: Dilute with a carrier oil (like coconut or jojoba oil) before applying to the skin. Use 1-2 drops of Tea Tree Oil per tablespoon of carrier oil.

- **Considerations**: Can be irritating if used undiluted. Avoid using near the eyes and on sensitive skin areas.

Herbal Beauty Treatments

Creating your own herbal beauty treatments at home can be rewarding and effective. Here are some simple and nourishing DIY recipes:

DIY Face Masks:

1. Hydrating Aloe Vera and Honey Mask:

- **Ingredients**: 2 tablespoons of Aloe Vera gel, 1 tablespoon of raw honey.

- **Preparation**: Mix the Aloe Vera gel and honey in a bowl until well combined.

- **Application**: Apply the mixture to your face, avoiding the eye area. Leave it on for 15-20 minutes before rinsing off with warm water.

- **Benefits**: This mask hydrates and soothes the skin, leaving it soft and glowing.

2. Anti-Acne Tea Tree and Green Clay Mask:

- **Ingredients**: 2 tablespoons of green clay, 3-4 drops of Tea Tree Oil, enough water or Aloe Vera gel to make a paste.

- **Preparation**: Mix the green clay and Tea Tree Oil. Add water or Aloe Vera gel to form a smooth paste.

- **Application**: Apply the mask to your face, avoiding the eye area. Leave it on for 10-15 minutes before rinsing off with warm water.

- **Benefits**: This mask helps absorb excess oil, unclog pores, and reduce acne breakouts.

3. Brightening Turmeric and Yogurt Mask:

- **Ingredients**: 1 teaspoon of turmeric powder, 2 tablespoons of plain yogurt.

- **Preparation**: Mix the turmeric powder and yogurt until well combined.

- **Application**: Apply the mixture to your face, avoiding the eye area. Leave it on for 10-15 minutes before rinsing off with warm water.

- **Benefits**: This mask brightens the complexion and reduces pigmentation and inflammation.

Herbal Infused Oils:

Herbal infused oils can be used for massage, moisturizing, and as a base for other skincare products.

1. Calendula Infused Oil:

- **Ingredients**: Dried calendula flowers, carrier oil (such as olive or jojoba oil).

- **Preparation**: Fill a jar with dried calendula flowers and cover with carrier oil. Seal the jar and place it in a sunny spot for 4-6 weeks, shaking occasionally. Strain the oil through a cheesecloth or fine mesh strainer and store it in a dark glass bottle.

- **Uses**: Use as a moisturizer, massage oil, or ingredient in homemade salves and lotions.

- **Benefits**: This oil is soothing, healing, and anti-inflammatory, perfect for sensitive or irritated skin.

2. Lavender Infused Oil:

- **Ingredients**: Dried lavender flowers, carrier oil (such as almond or grapeseed oil).

- **Preparation**: Fill a jar with dried lavender flowers and cover with carrier oil. Seal the jar and place it in a sunny spot for 4-6 weeks, shaking occasionally. Strain the oil through a cheesecloth or fine mesh strainer and store it in a dark glass bottle.

- **Uses**: Use as a calming massage oil, in baths, or as a moisturizer.

- **Benefits**: This oil is calming, soothing, and moisturizing, ideal for relaxing and nourishing the skin.

3. Chamomile Infused Oil:

- **Ingredients**: Dried chamomile flowers, carrier oil (such as sunflower or sweet almond oil).

- **Preparation**: Fill a jar with dried chamomile flowers and cover with carrier oil. Seal the jar and place it in a sunny spot for 4-6 weeks, shaking occasionally. Strain the oil through a cheesecloth or fine mesh strainer and store it in a dark glass bottle.

- **Uses**: Use as a soothing massage oil, in baths, or as a moisturizer.

- **Benefits**: This oil is soothing and anti-inflammatory, perfect for calming irritated or sensitive skin.

Herbal remedies offer a natural and effective approach to maintaining healthy, beautiful skin. By understanding common skin issues and their herbal solutions, and incorporating nourishing herbal treatments into your skincare routine, you can achieve a radiant and healthy complexion. Always consult with a healthcare provider or dermatologist before starting any new herbal regimen, especially if you have underlying skin conditions or are taking other medications. Embrace the power of nature to enhance your skin and beauty naturally.

Chapter 6:
Digestive Health and Detoxification
The Importance of Gut Health

Gut health is a cornerstone of overall well-being. The digestive system not only breaks down food and absorbs nutrients but also plays a crucial role in the immune system, hormone regulation, and mental health. Poor gut health can lead to a host of issues, including:

1. Digestive Disorders:

- **Irritable Bowel Syndrome (IBS)**: Characterized by abdominal pain, bloating, and altered bowel habits.

- **Inflammatory Bowel Disease (IBD)**: Includes Crohn's disease and ulcerative colitis, which cause chronic inflammation of the gastrointestinal tract.

- **Gastroesophageal Reflux Disease (GERD)**: A condition where stomach acid frequently flows back into the esophagus, causing heartburn and other symptoms.

2. Nutrient Deficiencies:

- Poor digestion and absorption can lead to deficiencies in essential vitamins and minerals, affecting overall health and vitality.

3. Immune Function:

- The gut houses a significant portion of the immune system. An imbalance in gut flora can weaken the immune response and increase susceptibility to infections.

4. Mental Health:

- The gut-brain axis is a communication network linking the gut and the brain. Gut health significantly impacts mood and mental health, with imbalances contributing to anxiety and depression.

5. Detoxification:

- The liver and kidneys, integral parts of the digestive system, are primary organs of detoxification. A healthy gut supports their function, facilitating the removal of toxins from the body.

Improving gut health involves a holistic approach, including dietary changes, stress management, and the use of beneficial herbs.

Herbs for Digestion

Herbs have been used for centuries to support digestive health. Here are some key herbs that can aid digestion and alleviate common digestive issues:

Peppermint (Mentha piperita):

- **Uses**: Peppermint is widely used to relieve symptoms of IBS, including abdominal pain, bloating, and gas. It also helps with indigestion and nausea.

- **Mechanism**: Contains menthol, which has antispasmodic properties that relax the muscles of the gastrointestinal tract and reduce spasms.

- **Preparation**: Consumed as a tea, capsule, or essential oil. For tea, steep 1-2 teaspoons of dried peppermint leaves in hot water for 10 minutes. Capsules containing enteric-coated peppermint oil are often used for IBS.

- **Considerations**: Generally safe for most people. Avoid peppermint oil in individuals with GERD as it may worsen symptoms.

Ginger (Zingiber officinale):

- **Uses**: Ginger is effective for nausea, vomiting, indigestion, and motion sickness.

It also helps stimulate digestion and reduce bloating.

- **Mechanism**: Contains gingerol and shogaol, compounds that enhance gastric motility, reduce inflammation, and relieve nausea.

- **Preparation**: Fresh ginger can be grated and added to foods or brewed as tea. Ginger capsules and tinctures are also available. For tea, steep 1-2 teaspoons of fresh grated ginger in hot water for 10-15 minutes.

- **Considerations**: Generally safe but may cause heartburn in some individuals. Consult a healthcare provider if you are pregnant or taking blood-thinning medications.

Fennel (Foeniculum vulgare):

- **Uses**: Fennel seeds are commonly used to relieve bloating, gas, and indigestion. They also help stimulate appetite and promote digestion.

- **Mechanism**: Contains anethole, which has carminative properties that help reduce gas and bloating by relaxing gastrointestinal muscles.

- **Preparation**: Consumed as a tea or chewed directly. For tea, steep 1-2 teaspoons of crushed fennel seeds in hot water for 10 minutes.

- **Considerations**: Generally safe for most people. Avoid if you have allergies to plants in the carrot family.

Detoxifying Herbs

Detoxifying herbs support the liver, kidneys, and other organs involved in the body's natural detoxification processes. Here are some key detoxifying herbs:

Dandelion (Taraxacum officinale):

- **Uses**: Dandelion root and leaves are used to support liver function, promote detoxification, and act as a diuretic to flush out toxins.

- **Mechanism**: Rich in vitamins and minerals, dandelion enhances bile production, aiding digestion and the elimination of toxins. It also has diuretic properties that increase urine output and help remove waste products.

- **Preparation**: Consumed as a tea, tincture, or capsule. For tea, steep 1-2 teaspoons of dried dandelion root or leaves in hot water for 10-15 minutes.

- **Considerations**: Generally safe for most people. Consult a healthcare provider if you have gallbladder issues or are taking diuretics.

Milk Thistle (Silybum marianum):

- **Uses**: Milk thistle is renowned for its liver-protective properties, helping to detoxify and regenerate liver cells.

- **Mechanism**: Contains silymarin, a compound that protects liver cells from toxins and promotes regeneration. It also has antioxidant and anti-inflammatory properties.

- **Preparation**: Available as a tea, tincture, or capsule. A typical dose is 200-400 mg of standardized silymarin extract daily.

- **Considerations**: Generally safe for most people. Consult a healthcare provider if you have a history of hormone-sensitive conditions.

Burdock Root (Arctium lappa):

- **Uses**: Burdock root is used to cleanse the blood, support liver function, and promote healthy skin.

- **Mechanism**: Contains inulin, a prebiotic fiber that supports gut health, and compounds that promote detoxification and have diuretic effects.

- **Preparation**: Consumed as a tea, tincture, or added to soups and stews. For tea, steep 1-2 teaspoons of dried burdock root in hot water for 10-15 minutes.

- **Considerations**: Generally safe for most people. Avoid if you have allergies to plants in the Asteraceae family.

Maintaining digestive health and supporting the body's natural detoxification processes are crucial for overall well-being. By incorporating herbs like peppermint, ginger, and fennel for digestion, and dandelion, milk thistle, and burdock root for detoxification, you can naturally enhance your digestive function and promote optimal health. Always consult with a healthcare provider before starting any new herbal regimen, especially if you have underlying health conditions or are taking other medications. Embrace the power of herbal remedies to support your gut health and detoxification naturally, fostering a healthier, more balanced life.

Chapter 7:
Herbal Support for Immune Health
Understanding the Immune System

The immune system is a complex network of cells, tissues, and organs that work together to defend the body against harmful pathogens, such as bacteria, viruses, and fungi. It plays a crucial role in maintaining health and preventing illness. The immune system can be broadly categorized into two main components:

1. Innate Immunity:

- **First Line of Defense**: Includes physical barriers like the skin and mucous membranes, as well as immune cells like phagocytes and natural killer cells.

- **Rapid Response**: Responds quickly to pathogens and does not require previous exposure to the invader.

2. Adaptive Immunity:

- **Specific Defense**: Involves lymphocytes (B cells and T cells) that recognize specific antigens and remember them for future attacks.

- **Slower Initial Response**: Takes longer to respond initially but provides long-lasting protection through immunological memory.

Key Immune System Functions:

- **Identification**: Detecting and recognizing pathogens.

- **Attack**: Mobilizing immune cells to destroy invaders.

- **Memory**: Remembering past infections to respond more quickly in the future.

- **Regulation**: Balancing immune responses to prevent overactivity (autoimmune diseases) or underactivity (immunodeficiency).

Maintaining a healthy immune system involves a balanced diet, regular exercise, adequate sleep, stress management, and, importantly, the support of immune-boosting herbs.

Herbs for Immune Support

Herbs have been used for centuries to enhance immune function and protect against infections. Here are some key herbs known for their immune-supportive properties:

Echinacea (Echinacea purpurea):

- **Uses**: Echinacea is widely used to prevent and treat upper respiratory infections, such as the common cold and flu. It also helps reduce the duration and severity of symptoms.

- **Mechanism**: Contains active compounds like alkamides, polysaccharides, and glycoproteins that stimulate immune cells, enhance phagocytosis, and increase the production of interferons.

- **Preparation**: Available as a tea, tincture, capsule, or extract. For tea, steep 1-2 teaspoons of dried Echinacea in hot water for 10-15 minutes. Tinctures are typically dosed at 2-4 ml, three times daily.

- **Considerations**: Generally safe for short-term use. Avoid if you have allergies to plants in the Asteraceae family or autoimmune disorders.

Elderberry (Sambucus nigra):

- **Uses**: Elderberry is used to prevent and treat viral infections, particularly influenza and colds. It has antiviral and immune-modulating properties.

- **Mechanism**: Rich in flavonoids, especially anthocyanins, which inhibit the replication of viruses and enhance the immune response. It also increases cytokine production, boosting immune activity.

- **Preparation**: Available as syrup, extract, capsule, or tea. For syrup, follow the dosage instructions on the product label. For tea, steep 1-2 teaspoons of dried elderberries in hot water for 10-15 minutes.

- **Considerations**: Generally safe when used properly. Raw elderberries contain toxic compounds and should always be cooked before consumption.

Astragalus (Astragalus membranaceus):

- **Uses**: Astragalus is used to enhance overall immune function, improve resistance to infections, and support recovery from illness.

- **Mechanism**: Contains saponins, flavonoids, and polysaccharides that stimulate immune cells, increase antibody production, and enhance antiviral activity.

- **Preparation**: Available as a tea, tincture, capsule, or extract. For tea, simmer 1-2 teaspoons of dried astragalus root in water for 20-30 minutes. Tinctures are typically dosed at 2-4 ml, three times daily.

- **Considerations**: Generally safe for long-term use. Avoid if you have autoimmune diseases or are taking immunosuppressant medications.

Preventative Herbal Strategies

In addition to using specific herbs for immune support, incorporating preventative herbal strategies can help maintain a robust immune system and reduce the risk of infections.

1. Herbal Teas and Tonics:

- **Daily Immune Tea**: Blend equal parts of Echinacea, elderberry, and astragalus with other supportive herbs like ginger and licorice. Drink daily to support immune health.

- **Fire Cider**: A traditional tonic made with apple cider vinegar infused with immune-boosting herbs and spices like garlic, ginger, horseradish, and cayenne pepper. Take 1-2 tablespoons daily as a preventative measure.

2. Adaptogenic Herbs:

- **Ashwagandha (Withania somnifera)**: Supports overall health, reduces stress, and enhances immune function.

- **Rhodiola (Rhodiola rosea)**: Helps the body adapt to stress, improves energy levels, and supports immune health.

- **Tulsi (Ocimum sanctum)**: Also known as Holy Basil, it helps reduce stress, support respiratory health, and boost immunity.

3. Nutritive Herbs:

- **Nettle (Urtica dioica)**: Rich in vitamins and minerals, supports overall health and vitality.

- **Oatstraw (Avena sativa)**: Provides essential nutrients and supports nervous system health.

4. Probiotic and Prebiotic Support:

- **Probiotics**: Beneficial bacteria that support gut health and immune function. Found in fermented foods like yogurt, kefir, sauerkraut, and kimchi.

- **Prebiotics**: Non-digestible fibers that feed beneficial gut bacteria. Found in foods like garlic, onions, leeks, asparagus, and bananas.

5. Lifestyle Practices:

- **Balanced Diet**: Emphasize whole, nutrient-dense foods rich in vitamins, minerals, and antioxidants. Include plenty of fruits, vegetables, whole grains, lean proteins, and healthy fats.

- **Regular Exercise**: Engage in moderate physical activity to boost circulation, reduce stress, and support immune function.

- **Adequate Sleep**: Aim for 7-9 hours of quality sleep each night to allow the body to rest and repair.

- **Stress Management**: Practice stress-reducing techniques like meditation, yoga, deep breathing, and spending time in nature.

- **Good Hygiene**: Wash hands regularly, avoid touching your face, and maintain a clean living environment to reduce the risk of infections.

Supporting the immune system with herbal remedies and preventative strategies is an effective way to maintain health and prevent illness. By incorporating immune-boosting herbs like Echinacea, elderberry, and astragalus into your daily routine, along with adaptogenic and nutritive herbs, you can strengthen your body's natural defenses. Additionally, adopting a healthy lifestyle, rich in nutritious foods, regular exercise, adequate sleep, and stress management, will further enhance your immune health. Always consult with a healthcare provider before starting any new herbal regimen, especially if you have underlying health conditions or are taking other medications. Embrace the power of nature to support your immune system and overall well-being naturally.

Chapter 8:
Mental Clarity and Cognitive Health
Herbal Nootropics

Nootropics are substances that enhance cognitive function, particularly executive functions, memory, creativity, or motivation, in healthy individuals. Herbal nootropics have been used traditionally to improve mental clarity, focus, and cognitive health. Here are some key herbal nootropics:

Ginkgo Biloba (Ginkgo biloba):

- **Uses**: Ginkgo Biloba is widely used to enhance memory, improve cognitive function, and increase mental alertness. It is also known for its potential to help with age-related cognitive decline and conditions such as dementia and Alzheimer's disease.

- **Mechanism**: Ginkgo biloba contains flavonoids and terpenoids, which have antioxidant properties that protect nerve cells. It improves blood flow to the brain and enhances neural plasticity.

- **Preparation**: Available as capsules, tablets, tinctures, and teas. The recommended dose is typically 120-240 mg per day of standardized extract, divided into two or three doses.

- **Considerations**: Generally safe for most people. However, it can interact with blood-thinning medications and increase the risk of bleeding.

Bacopa Monnieri (Bacopa monnieri):

- **Uses**: Bacopa Monnieri, also known as Brahmi, is used to improve memory, learning, and concentration. It has adaptogenic properties that help reduce anxiety and stress.

- **Mechanism**: Contains bacosides, which enhance communication between neurons, repair damaged neurons, and protect brain cells from oxidative stress. It also increases the levels of neurotransmitters such as serotonin.

- **Preparation**: Available as capsules, tablets, powders, and tinctures. The recommended dose is typically 300-450 mg per day of standardized extract containing 50% bacosides.

- **Considerations**: Generally safe for most people. Some individuals may experience digestive discomfort. Consult a healthcare provider if you are pregnant, breastfeeding, or taking medications.

Gotu Kola (Centella asiatica):

- **Uses**: Gotu Kola is used to enhance cognitive function, improve memory, and promote mental clarity. It is also known for its calming effects and ability to reduce anxiety.

- **Mechanism**: Contains triterpenoids, which enhance cognitive function by promoting neurogenesis and synaptic plasticity. It also improves blood circulation to the brain and has antioxidant properties.

- **Preparation**: Available as capsules, tablets, tinctures, and teas. The recommended dose is typically 500-1000 mg of dried herb or 30-60 drops of tincture per day.

- **Considerations**: Generally safe for most people. Some individuals may experience headaches or dizziness. Avoid if you are pregnant, breastfeeding, or have liver disease.

Essential Oils for Focus and Memory

Essential oils are highly concentrated plant extracts that can support cognitive function through their aromatic properties. Here are some essential oils known to enhance focus and memory:

Rosemary (Rosmarinus officinalis):

- **Uses**: Rosemary essential oil is used to improve concentration, enhance memory, and increase mental alertness. It is also known for its uplifting and invigorating effects.

- **Mechanism**: Contains compounds such as 1,8-cineole and camphor, which stimulate the central nervous system and improve blood flow to the brain. Aromatic inhalation of rosemary essential oil can enhance cognitive performance and mood.

- **Preparation**: Use in aromatherapy diffusers, apply topically (diluted in a carrier oil), or inhale directly from the bottle. Add 3-5 drops to a diffuser or mix with a carrier oil for topical application.

- **Considerations**: Generally safe for most people. Avoid during pregnancy and do not use on infants or young children. Always dilute before topical use.

Peppermint (Mentha piperita):

- **Uses**: Peppermint essential oil is used to improve focus, enhance mental clarity, and increase alertness. It has a refreshing and stimulating aroma that can help reduce mental fatigue.

- **Mechanism**: Contains menthol, which has stimulating effects on the brain and can improve cognitive performance and memory. It also enhances blood circulation and oxygenation to the brain.

- **Preparation**: Use in aromatherapy diffusers, apply topically (diluted in a carrier oil), or inhale directly from the bottle. Add 3-5 drops to a diffuser or mix with a carrier oil for topical application.

- **Considerations**: Generally safe for most people. Avoid use in children under 6 years old and always dilute before topical use. May cause skin irritation in sensitive individuals.

Lemon Balm (Melissa officinalis):

- **Uses**: Lemon balm essential oil is used to improve cognitive function, enhance memory, and promote relaxation. It has calming and uplifting effects that can help reduce anxiety and improve mood.

- **Mechanism**: Contains compounds such as rosmarinic acid and citral, which have neuroprotective and antioxidant properties.

It also modulates neurotransmitter activity, enhancing cognitive performance and reducing stress.

- **Preparation**: Use in aromatherapy diffusers, apply topically (diluted in a carrier oil), or inhale directly from the bottle. Add 3-5 drops to a diffuser or mix with a carrier oil for topical application.

- **Considerations**: Generally safe for most people. Avoid use in children under 6 years old and always dilute before topical use. May cause skin irritation in sensitive individuals.

Integrating Herbal and Aromatic Strategies

Combining herbal nootropics and essential oils can provide a comprehensive approach to enhancing mental clarity and cognitive health. Here are some strategies to integrate these natural remedies into your daily routine:

1. Morning Routine:

- **Herbal Tea**: Start your day with a cup of herbal tea made from a blend of ginkgo biloba, bacopa monnieri, and gotu kola. This can help boost cognitive function and mental clarity for the day ahead.

- **Essential Oil Diffusion**: Use a diffuser with rosemary and peppermint essential oils in your workspace or home office to enhance focus and alertness.

2. Study or Work Sessions:

- **Herbal Supplements**: Take standardized extracts of ginkgo biloba, bacopa monnieri, or gotu kola as supplements to support cognitive performance and memory.

- **Inhalation Techniques**: Keep a bottle of peppermint or rosemary essential oil at your desk. Inhale deeply from the bottle or apply a diluted drop to your wrists to boost concentration and reduce mental fatigue.

3. Evening Routine:

- **Calming Tea**: In the evening, enjoy a cup of lemon balm tea to promote relaxation and improve sleep quality. This can help reduce stress and enhance cognitive function the next day.

- **Aromatic Relaxation**: Diffuse lemon balm essential oil in your bedroom or use it in a relaxing bath before bedtime to unwind and prepare for restful sleep.

4. Stress Management:

- **Adaptogenic Herbs**: Incorporate adaptogenic herbs like ashwagandha and rhodiola into your routine to reduce stress and support cognitive health.

- **Mindfulness Practices**: Combine the use of essential oils with mindfulness practices such as meditation or deep breathing exercises to enhance mental clarity and reduce stress.

Supporting mental clarity and cognitive health with herbal nootropics and essential oils can be a natural and effective approach to enhancing brain function. By incorporating herbs like ginkgo biloba, bacopa monnieri, and gotu kola, along with essential oils like rosemary, peppermint, and lemon balm, you can improve focus, memory, and overall cognitive performance. Always consult with a healthcare provider before starting any new herbal or essential oil regimen, especially if you have underlying health conditions or are taking other medications. Embrace the power of natural remedies to support your cognitive health and enhance your mental clarity.

Chapter 9:
Herbal Remedies for Reproductive Health

Fertility-Boosting Herbs

Fertility is a complex aspect of reproductive health influenced by various factors, including hormonal balance, ovulation, sperm quality, and overall health. Herbal remedies have been used for centuries to support fertility and increase the chances of conception. Here are some key fertility-boosting herbs:

Red Raspberry Leaf (Rubus idaeus):

- **Uses**: Red raspberry leaf is known as a uterine tonic, supporting overall reproductive health. It is often used to tone the uterus in preparation for conception and pregnancy.

- **Mechanism**: Contains fragarine, an alkaloid that helps strengthen and tone the muscles of the uterus, improving its function. It also contains vitamins and minerals that support fertility.

- **Preparation**: Consumed as a tea or in capsule form. For tea, steep 1-2 teaspoons of dried red raspberry leaves in hot water for 10-15 minutes.

- **Considerations**: Generally safe for most people. Avoid high doses during early pregnancy.

Shatavari (Asparagus racemosus):

- **Uses**: Shatavari is revered in Ayurvedic medicine as a rejuvenating herb for female reproductive health. It supports hormonal balance, nourishes the reproductive organs, and enhances fertility.

- **Mechanism**: Contains saponins and phytoestrogens that regulate hormonal levels, particularly estrogen, promoting ovulation and supporting the menstrual cycle. It also has adaptogenic properties that help reduce stress.

- **Preparation**: Available as a powder, capsule, or tincture. The recommended dose is typically 500-1000 mg of powder or 30-60 drops of tincture daily.

- **Considerations**: Generally safe for most people. Avoid during pregnancy without consulting a healthcare provider.

Nettle (Urtica dioica):

- **Uses**: Nettle is a nutritive herb rich in vitamins, minerals, and antioxidants. It supports overall health and may enhance fertility by providing essential nutrients.

- **Mechanism**: Contains vitamins A, C, and K, as well as minerals like iron, calcium, and magnesium, which are important for reproductive health. It also has detoxifying properties that support liver function.

- **Preparation**: Consumed as a tea, infusion, or in cooked dishes. For tea, steep 1-2 teaspoons of dried nettle leaves in hot water for 10-15 minutes.

- **Considerations**: Generally safe for most people. Avoid excessive consumption due to its diuretic effects.

Herbs for Pregnancy and Postpartum

Pregnancy and postpartum are critical periods in a woman's reproductive journey, requiring special care and support. Herbal remedies can play a valuable role in promoting a healthy pregnancy, supporting the mother's well-being, and aiding postpartum recovery. Here are some key herbs for pregnancy and postpartum:

Ginger (Zingiber officinale):

- **Uses**: Ginger is commonly used to alleviate nausea and vomiting during pregnancy, especially morning sickness. It also aids digestion and reduces inflammation.

- **Mechanism**: Contains gingerol and shogaol, compounds that help soothe the stomach and alleviate nausea. Ginger also has antioxidant and anti-inflammatory properties.

- **Preparation**: Consumed as tea, capsules, or fresh ginger. For tea, steep 1-2 teaspoons of fresh grated ginger in hot water for 10-15 minutes.

- **Considerations**: Generally safe for most pregnant women when used in moderate amounts. Consult a healthcare provider if you have pregnancy-related complications.

Oat Straw (Avena sativa):

- **Uses**: Oat straw is rich in nutrients and has nervine properties that support the nervous system and promote relaxation. It is beneficial during pregnancy and postpartum for reducing stress and anxiety.

- **Mechanism**: Contains B vitamins, minerals, and compounds like avenanthramides, which have calming effects on the nervous system. Oat straw helps reduce stress and support emotional well-being.

- **Preparation**: Consumed as a tea, infusion, or tincture. For tea, steep 1-2 teaspoons of dried oat straw in hot water for 10-15 minutes.

- **Considerations**: Generally safe for most pregnant and breastfeeding women. Avoid if you have gluten sensitivity or celiac disease.

Fenugreek (Trigonella foenum-graecum):

- **Uses**: Fenugreek is known for its galactagogue properties, promoting lactation and milk production in breastfeeding mothers. It can also help regulate blood sugar levels and support postpartum recovery.

- **Mechanism**: Contains compounds like diosgenin and galactomannan, which stimulate milk production by increasing prolactin levels. Fenugreek also has anti-inflammatory and antioxidant effects.

- **Preparation**: Consumed as capsules, tea, or seeds. For tea, steep 1-2 teaspoons of fenugreek seeds in hot water for 10-15 minutes.

- **Considerations**: Generally safe for most breastfeeding women when used in moderate amounts. Avoid if you have allergies to plants in the Fabaceae family.

Integrating Herbal Support into Reproductive Health

Incorporating herbal remedies into your reproductive health regimen can provide natural support throughout your journey, from preconception to postpartum. Here are some strategies to integrate herbal support into your routine:

1. Preconception Care:

- **Herbal Blends**: Create personalized herbal blends combining fertility-boosting herbs like red raspberry leaf, shatavari, and nettle to support reproductive health and prepare the body for conception.

- **Nutritional Support**: Incorporate nutrient-rich foods and supplements to optimize fertility, including vitamins, minerals, and omega-3 fatty acids.

2. Pregnancy Support:

- **Nausea Relief**: Use ginger tea or capsules to alleviate nausea and vomiting during pregnancy. Peppermint and lemon balm teas can also help soothe an upset stomach.

- **Nutritive Infusions**: Drink nourishing infusions of oat straw or nettle throughout pregnancy to support overall health and provide essential nutrients for both mother and baby.

3. Postpartum Recovery:

- **Lactation Support**: Consume fenugreek tea or capsules to promote milk production and support breastfeeding. Fenugreek can also aid in postpartum hormone regulation and recovery.

- **Emotional Well-being**: Incorporate calming herbs like oat straw and chamomile into your postpartum routine to reduce stress, anxiety, and promote relaxation.

Herbal remedies offer valuable support for reproductive health, from enhancing fertility and supporting pregnancy to aiding postpartum recovery. By incorporating fertility-boosting herbs like red raspberry leaf, shatavari, and nettle into preconception care, and utilizing herbs like ginger, oat straw, and fenugreek during pregnancy and postpartum, women can naturally support their reproductive journey. Always consult with a healthcare provider before starting any new herbal regimen, especially if you have underlying health conditions or are pregnant or breastfeeding.

Embrace the power of herbal remedies to promote reproductive health and well-being naturally.

Chapter 10:
Creating Your Own Herbal Apothecary

Essential Tools and Supplies

Building your herbal apothecary requires a few essential tools and supplies to prepare and store herbal remedies effectively. Here are some must-have items:

1. Mortar and Pestle: Used for grinding herbs into powder or crushing them to release their medicinal properties.

2. Glass Jars and Bottles: Essential for storing dried herbs, tinctures, infusions, and other herbal preparations. Choose dark-colored glass to protect herbs from light exposure.

3. Stainless Steel Strainer or Cheesecloth: Used for straining herbal infusions, decoctions, and tinctures to remove plant material.

4. Double Boiler or Bain-Marie: Essential for gently heating herbs in oils or beeswax to make salves and balms without burning them.

5. Measuring Spoons and Cups: Accurate measurement is crucial for preparing herbal remedies with consistency and precision.

6. Labeling Supplies: Use waterproof labels and a permanent marker to label your herbal preparations with the herb used, date of preparation, and dosage instructions.

7. Storage Containers: Apart from glass jars, consider having small containers for storing herbal salves, balms, and creams.

Sourcing and Storing Herbs

Selecting high-quality herbs is essential for the efficacy and safety of your herbal remedies. Here are some tips for sourcing and storing herbs:

1. Sourcing:

- **Local Herb Shops**: Support local herb shops and apothecaries that specialize in organic, sustainably sourced herbs.

- **Online Suppliers**: Choose reputable online suppliers that provide detailed information about the sourcing, harvesting, and processing of their herbs.

- **Wildcrafting**: Harvesting herbs ethically and sustainably from your garden or the wild requires knowledge and respect for the environment and local regulations.

2. Storing:

- **Cool, Dark, and Dry**: Store dried herbs in airtight containers in a cool, dark, and dry place to preserve their potency and freshness.

- **Labeling**: Label each container with the herb's name, date of purchase or harvest, and any specific instructions for storage or use.

- **Rotation**: Regularly rotate your herb stock to ensure freshness and potency. Discard any herbs that show signs of mold, moisture, or insect infestation.

Basic Recipes and Preparations

Mastering basic herbal preparations allows you to create a wide range of remedies for various health concerns. Here are some essential recipes and preparations:

1. Tinctures:

- **Ingredients**: Dried herbs, alcohol (such as vodka or brandy), glass jar with lid.

- **Process**: Fill a glass jar with dried herbs and cover with alcohol. Seal the jar and let it sit for 4-6 weeks, shaking it daily. Strain the tincture and store in glass bottles.

- **Dosage**: Typically, 30-60 drops diluted in water, taken 2-3 times per day.

2. Infusions and Decoctions:

- **Ingredients**: Dried herbs, water, stainless steel pot with lid.

- **Infusions**: Pour boiling water over dried herbs, cover, and steep for 10-15 minutes. Strain and drink as a tea.

- **Decoctions**: Simmer herbs in water for 20-30 minutes, then strain. Decoctions are used for tougher plant parts like roots, bark, and seeds.

3. Herbal Salves and Balms:

- **Ingredients**: Dried herbs, carrier oil (such as olive oil or coconut oil), beeswax, essential oils (optional).

- **Process**: Infuse herbs in oil using the double boiler method, strain, and mix with melted beeswax. Add essential oils if desired. Pour into containers and let it cool and solidify.

Integrating Herbal Remedies into Your Lifestyle

Incorporating herbal remedies into your daily life can support overall health and well-being. Here are some ways to integrate herbal remedies into your lifestyle:

1. Morning Rituals: Start your day with a cup of herbal tea or a few drops of a tincture to boost energy, focus, or immunity.

2. Self-Care Practices: Use herbal-infused oils or balms for massage, skincare, or relaxation rituals to nourish the body and calm the mind.

3. Culinary Adventures: Experiment with incorporating culinary herbs into your meals and recipes to add flavor and therapeutic benefits.

4. Herbal First Aid Kit: Prepare a herbal first aid kit with remedies for common ailments like colds, headaches, cuts, and bruises.

5. Mindful Moments: Take moments throughout the day to pause, breathe deeply, and connect with the healing power of plants through aromatherapy or herbal teas.

Creating your own herbal apothecary is a rewarding and empowering journey that allows you to harness the healing power of plants for yourself and your loved ones. By equipping yourself with essential tools and supplies, sourcing and storing high-quality herbs, mastering basic recipes and preparations, and integrating herbal remedies into your lifestyle, you can cultivate a deeper connection with nature and support your health and well-being naturally. Embrace the art and science of herbalism as you

embark on this transformative journey of self-care
and healing.

84

Conclusion

As you embark on your journey with herbal remedies, it's essential to integrate them seamlessly into your daily life, finding balance and vitality naturally. By incorporating these botanical allies into your routines and rituals, you can tap into their healing potential and support your overall well-being. Here are some key points to keep in mind as you continue on this path:

Integrating Herbal Remedies into Daily Life

Embrace herbal remedies as a part of your daily life, weaving them into your routines and rituals. Start your day with a cup of herbal tea, use herbal-infused oils for self-massage or skincare, and turn to herbal tinctures or salves for common ailments. By incorporating herbal remedies into your daily routines, you can experience their benefits on a consistent basis and cultivate a deeper connection with nature.

Finding Balance and Vitality Naturally

Herbal remedies offer a holistic approach to health and wellness, supporting the body's natural ability to heal and thrive. As you explore different herbs and preparations, listen to your body's signals and find what works best for you. Remember that balance is key, and it's essential to nourish not just the physical body but also the mind, heart, and spirit. Cultivate practices that promote balance, vitality, and resilience in all aspects of your life.

Resources for Further Learning

Continued learning is an essential aspect of herbalism, as there is always more to discover and explore. Seek out reputable books, courses, and workshops to deepen your knowledge and understanding of herbal medicine. Connect with herbalists, community herbalism groups, and online forums to share experiences, ask questions, and learn from others' wisdom. By continually expanding your herbal knowledge, you can become more confident and empowered in using herbal remedies for yourself and others.

Final Thoughts and Encouragement

Embarking on a journey with herbal remedies is both a personal and transformative experience. As you explore the vast world of plants and their healing properties, trust in your intuition and embrace the wisdom of nature. Remember that herbal medicine is a gentle and supportive modality that works best in conjunction with a healthy lifestyle, including nutritious diet, regular exercise, adequate rest, and stress management. Trust in the healing power of plants and the innate wisdom of

your body as you journey towards greater health
and vitality.